NO GALLBLADDER DIET COOKBOOK

FOR BEGINNERS

QUICK AND EASY RECIPES FOR DIGESTION AFTER THE REMOVAL OF GALLBLADDER

IVAN ERICA

Table of Contents

UNDERSTANDING THE GALLBLADDER

The Gallbladder's function in digestion

Though it may not be as visible as the heart or the brain, the gallbladder is a tiny pear-shaped organ that is nestled beneath the liver and is extremely important to our digestive system. Its main job is to store and concentrate bile, the liver's yellow-brown digesting enzyme. The process of breaking down and absorbing lipids in the small intestine is made easier by bile and is crucial to the equilibrium and well-being of our bodies.

Bile salts, cholesterol, bilirubin, and other chemicals make up bile. Bile is continuously produced by the liver, passes through the bile ducts, and is kept in reserve in the gallbladder. The gallbladder contracts when we eat foods high in fat, causing bile to be released into the small intestine. Here, bile salts perform a process called emulsification, which breaks down the big fat molecules into smaller ones. Because it increases the surface area of lipids, this breakdown is essential because it makes them more accessible to digestive enzymes and facilitates their absorption into the bloodstream.

There is more to the gallbladder's role in digestion than just emulsifying fats. It also guarantees the efficient absorption of vital fatty acids and fat-soluble vitamins (A, D, E, and K). Our body would find it difficult to absorb these vital nutrients without the gallbladder's help, which could result in deficits and health problems.

Cholecystectomy, the removal of the gallbladder, is a common treatment that is frequently carried out as a result of gallstones or other gallbladder problems. The gallbladder is an organ that the body can survive without, but its absence affects the digestive system. The liver must immediately discharge bile into the small intestine in the absence of a storage space. When digesting significant amounts of fats, the gallbladder's concentrated bursts of bile can be more effective than this continuous trickle.

Following a cholecystectomy, people may suffer changes in their digestion and need to modify their diet. The "No Gallbladder Diet Cookbook for Beginners" is intended to serve as a reference for people who have had this surgery. The recipes in this book are designed to facilitate digestion by using simpler-to-digest items and reducing fat content to make up for the gallbladder's inability to store bile.

The gallbladder may be tiny, yet it plays a big part in digestion. Knowing the purpose of this organ enables us to better appreciate the intricate dance of bodily functions that takes place each time we eat. It's critical for people without gallbladders to adjust to dietary changes in order to preserve their general health and digestive tract. The goal of this book is to give readers a thorough guide to scrumptious, gallbladder-friendly dishes that promote a happy, balanced diet.

Effect of Gallbladder Removal

Cholecystectomy, the technical term for the removal of the gallbladder, is a procedure that can significantly impact a person's digestive system and general health. This chapter explores the effects of losing this little but vital organ and how it affects the body's capacity to digest food.

A cholecystectomy is frequently carried out to treat gallstones, inflammation, or other problems pertaining to the gallbladder. Although the procedure is usually safe and fixes the acute issues brought on by a sick gallbladder, it requires a lifetime of dietary and digestive adjustments.

Following the removal of their gallbladder, patients may experience symptoms like bloating, abdominal pain, and changes in bowel patterns. Usually transient, these symptoms get better as the body adjusts to not having the gallbladder.

Bile enters the small intestine straight from the liver in the absence of a gallbladder. Bile acid diarrhoea or bile acid malabsorption are conditions that might result from this continuous dripping of bile. It happens when bile acids build up in the colon rather than being properly reabsorbed, which causes loose stools and urgency.

The way lipids are absorbed is also impacted by the lack of the gallbladder. People may find it difficult to digest significant amounts of fat, which can result in symptoms like indigestion and diarrhoea, as bile is no longer generated in reaction to fatty meals. Consequently, low-fat diets are frequently advised.

It takes knowledge of which meals to include and which to avoid in order to adjust to living without a gallbladder. Eat fattening items in moderation, such as fatty meat cuts, full-fat dairy products, and fried dishes. Rather, a diet high in fruits, vegetables, whole grains, and lean meats can support the maintenance of a healthy digestive tract.

In order to maintain digestive health after a cholecystectomy, fibre is essential. Foods high in soluble fibre, such as beans, apples, and oats, can aid in the binding of bile acids and lessen the signs and symptoms of bile acid malabsorption. Whole grains and vegetables include insoluble fibre, which promotes regular bowel motions and staves against constipation.

For those without a gallbladder, it is imperative to keep a careful eye on their symptoms and dietary reactions. Maintaining a food journal might assist in identifying trigger foods and eating habits that make digestive problems worse. Consulting with a dietician or nutritionist can also offer individualised advice and assistance.

Because of the substantial implications of gallbladder removal, diet and nutrition must be carefully considered. People can live a healthy and pleasant life without a gallbladder by being aware of the changes in digestion and modifying their food habits accordingly.

Adating to life without Gallbladder

Many people have to live without a gallbladder, and while it can be intimidating at first, learning how to modify your food and way of living can help you live a long and healthy life. The modifications and factors to be taken into account in order to control digestion and preserve health following gallbladder removal are the major topic of this chapter.

The human body has remarkable adaptability, and it starts adjusting to the new digestive mechanism immediately after the gallbladder is removed. The liver now sends bile straight into the small intestine from where it was formerly concentrated and kept in the gallbladder. Bile is still there to help with fat digestion as a result of this alteration, but it is less concentrated and less easily accessible in big quantities when needed. Consequently, people without a gallbladder must watch how much fat they eat.

Dietary adjustments are the most important modification for people without a gallbladder. A diet low in fat is frequently advised to reduce the chance of experiencing stomach discomfort. dishes heavy in fat, like processed snacks, fried dishes, and fatty meats, should be eaten in moderation. Rather than overburdening the digestive system, a diet abundant in fruits, vegetables, lean meats, and whole grains can supply the essential elements.

Planning your meals becomes crucial for maintaining your nutrition after a cholecystectomy. Having smaller, more frequent meals instead of larger, more uncomfortable ones will assist guarantee a consistent supply of bile for digestion. Making meals at home gives you more control over the fat and food level, which makes it simpler to follow a diet that is friendly to your gallbladder.

Making healthy decisions can be aided by knowing the various types of fats as not all fats are made equal. Healthy fats that can be incorporated into the diet in moderation are monounsaturated and polyunsaturated fats, which are present in foods like avocados, almonds, and fish. Limiting trans and saturated fats, which are frequently included in baked products and fast meals, is recommended.

Because it can aid in the binding of bile acids and lessen the symptoms of bile acid malabsorption, soluble fibre is advantageous for people without a gallbladder. Soluble fiber-rich foods, like oats, lentils, and some fruits, can facilitate better digestion and help control bowel motions.

Maintaining regular physical activity and drinking plenty of water are also crucial for digestive health. Exercise can assist to accelerate digestion and reduce constipation, while water can help flush the system and aid in the digestion and absorption of nutrients.

It takes time to learn about your body's new requirements and how to carefully respond in order to adjust to living without a gallbladder

NUTRITIONAL FOUNDATION

Macronutrients and Micronutrients

Setting out on a voyage without a gallbladder requires a more thorough comprehension of the components that comprise the foundation of our diet. The goal of this chapter is to provide readers with a foundation for making educated dietary decisions that promote healthy digestion and general health by demystifying the complicated world of macronutrients and micronutrients.

Macronutrients: The Fuel for the Body
As our body's main source of energy, macronutrients are the nutrients we need in big quantities. They consist of lipids, proteins, and carbohydrates, each of which has a special function in preserving biological processes.

Carbohydrates: A vital source of energy, carbohydrates are sometimes misinterpreted. Fruits, vegetables, grains, and legumes all contain them. Due to their high fibre content, complex carbohydrates are especially good for people without gallbladders since they support healthy digestion and offer a consistent release of energy.

Proteins: Essential for tissue growth and repair, proteins are the building blocks of life. For people who have had their gallbladder removed, lean proteins like chicken, fish, tofu, and beans are great options because they are high in vital amino acids but low in fat.

Fats: Although those without gallbladders should exercise caution when consuming fats, it's vital to keep in mind that not all fats are harmful. Small levels of monounsaturated and polyunsaturated fats, which are present in avocados, nuts, and some oils, can help maintain heart health and cell function.

Micronutrients: Essential to Overall Health
Micronutrients are vitamins and minerals that are needed in lower amounts and are essential for many body functions.

Vitamins: These natural substances are essential for development, immunity, and general well-being. Following a cholecystectomy, fat-soluble vitamins (A, D, E, and K) are especially important because of potential absorption issues. To assist ensure proper intake, include a variety of fruits and vegetables in your diet.

Minerals: Vital minerals that support nerve function, fluid balance, and bone health include calcium, potassium, and magnesium. Nuts, leafy greens, and dairy substitutes are excellent providers of these vital nutrients.

Nutrient Balancing Without a Gallbladder
Managing a diet without a gallbladder requires an understanding of the balance and interactions between macronutrients and micronutrients. It's important to create harmony in your meals rather than merely cutting fat if you want to make sure that all of your nutritional demands are satisfied without causing intestinal irritation.

The yin and yang of nutrition are macronutrients and micronutrients, each of which contributes to the maintenance of life and the advancement of health. Paying special attention to these nutrients can result in a balanced diet that improves quality of life and aids in digestion for people who do not have a gallbladder.

The cornerstone of excellent health is a balanced diet, particularly for people who have had their gallbladder removed. The importance of sustaining a diet that balances all food categories is discussed in this part in order to guarantee that the body gets the nutrients it requires to operate at its best.

A well-balanced diet is like a masterfully composed symphony, with every nutrient performing its part in perfect harmony with all the others. This balance is even more important for those without a gallbladder because it can have a major impact on their digestion and general health.

Food Groups

A diverse range of foods from each of the five main food groups are part of a balanced diet:

Fruits and Vegetables: These should make up half of your plate because they are high in fibre, vitamins, and minerals. They support digestive health and offer a variety of nutrients necessary for post-surgery maintenance and rehabilitation.

Grains: A quarter of your dish should consist of entire grains. They are a great source of energy and provide fibre, which helps with digestion and may help prevent problems like bile acid diarrhoea that may arise after a cholecystectomy.

Proteins: A quarter of your dish need to be made up of lean proteins. They are necessary for maintaining muscular mass and mending tissues. Fish, chicken, beans, and nuts are among the best options because they supply you the essential proteins without being overly fattening.

Dairy: Calcium and vitamin D, which are essential for healthy bones, can be found in low-fat or fat-free dairy products. Almond or soy milk are good options for people who are lactose intolerant or trying to cut back on their fat consumption.

Fats: Although people without a gallbladder should consume less fat, good fats are still essential for brain function and nutrition absorption. In moderation, sources such as avocados, seeds, and olive oil can be included.

Moderation and variety are the cornerstones of a balanced diet. Consuming a diverse array of meals guarantees that you receive a range of nutrients, and consuming any one food type in moderation helps avoid overindulging, especially fats, which can be more difficult to digest after a cholecystectomy.

Maintaining a balanced diet can be facilitated by the practice of mindful eating. It entails paying close attention to the body's signals of hunger and fullness, appreciating every bite, and being totally present throughout meals. This might assist detect foods that might cause discomfort and reduce overeating.

One cannot stress the value of eating a balanced diet, particularly for people getting used to living without a gallbladder. People can support their digestive systems and advance their general health by making sure their meals are nutrient-dense and well-rounded.

Reading Food Labels

It can be difficult to navigate the world of diet, particularly for people who are getting used to living without a gallbladder. Comprehending food labels is a crucial ability that can enable people to make better decisions and have a balanced diet. You will learn about the essential components of food labels in this part, along with what to look for to fulfil your dietary requirements.

One useful tool for determining the nutritional value of food products is the Nutrition Facts panel seen on food packaging. Here are some things to consider:

Serving Size: Prioritise determining the serving size. It serves as the foundation for the nutritional data offered and varies greatly throughout goods.

Calories: The amount of energy you receive from food is indicated by the number of calories per serving. People without gallbladders should watch how many calories they consume overall, especially from fats.

Macronutrients: Consider the following: total fat, cholesterol, sodium, trans fat, saturated fat, sugars, and protein. It's especially crucial to watch fat intake after a cholecystectomy to prevent stomach discomfort.

%Daily Values: These numbers give you an idea of how much of each nutrient a serving of a food adds to your daily intake. Aim for lower percentages of fat, cholesterol, and sodium and higher percentages of dietary fibre, vitamins, and minerals.

List of Ingredients
The nutrition information is not nearly as significant as the ingredients list. The product's ingredients are arranged in descending order of weight, with the most common elements being listed first.
entire Foods: Seek for goods that identify entire foods—like fruits, vegetables, or whole grains as the primary ingredient.
Additives: Take care when using additives, such as artificial sweeteners, colours, flavours, and preservatives. These can occasionally cause stomach problems, particularly in those who are sensitive.

Hidden Fats: Keep in mind that oils and creams are examples of hidden fat sources that might cause issues for people who don't have a gallbladder.

Medical Claims
Health claims are frequently found on food packaging, and they can be deceptive as well as useful. It's critical to comprehend the true implications of these statements.

"Low-Fat" and "Fat-Free": These designations denote a product's lower fat level, although it's possible that it still has a sizable sugar and other additive content.

Reduced Sodium: This means that although the product has less sodium than the original, its overall sodium content may still be excessive.

High in Fibre:This is a desired claim for people without a gallbladder because fibre helps regulate bile acid malabsorption and facilitate digestion.

One essential skill that can help you make wise eating choices is reading food labels. Knowing what foods contain and how they are made will help you choose foods that will best suit your needs after having your gallbladder removed.

BREAKFAST RECIPES

AVOCADO TOAST WITH POACHED EGG

**Time Required:
10 Minutes**

———————————

Servings: 1

Ingredients:

- slice whole-grain bread
- 1/2 ripe avocado
- 1 egg
- Salt and pepper to taste
- Fresh herbs (optional)

Instructions:

- Toast the bread to your liking.
- Mash the avocado and spread it on the toast.
- Poach the egg in simmering water for 3-4 minutes.
- Place the poached egg on top of the avocado toast.
- Season with salt, pepper, and fresh herbs if desired.

BERRY AND CHIA YOGURT PARFAIT

**Time Required:
5 Minutes**

———————————

Servings: 1

Ingredients:

- 1 cup low-fat Greek yogurt
- 1/2 cup mixed berries (strawberries, blueberries, raspberries)
- 2 tablespoons chia seeds
- 1 tablespoon honey (optional)

Instructions:

- In a glass, layer half of the yogurt.
- Add a layer of mixed berries.
- Sprinkle 1 tablespoon of chia seeds.
- Repeat the layers.
- Drizzle with honey if desired.

OATMEAL WITH ALMOND MILK AND NUTS

**Time Required:
15 Minutes**

____

Servings: 1

Ingredients:

- 1/2 cup rolled oats
- 1 cup almond milk
- 1 tablespoon almonds, chopped
- 1 tablespoon walnuts, chopped
- Cinnamon to taste

Instructions:

- Cook oats with almond milk according to package instructions.
- Once cooked, transfer to a bowl.
- Top with chopped almonds, walnuts, and a sprinkle of cinnamon.

SPINACH AND MUSHROOM OMELETTE

**Time Required:
15 Minutes**

____

Servings: 1

Ingredients:

- 2 egg whites
- 1/2 cup spinach, chopped
- 1/4 cup mushrooms, sliced
- Salt and pepper to taste
- Cooking spray

Instructions:

- Heat a non-stick pan and lightly coat with cooking spray.
- Sauté mushrooms until soft.
- Add spinach and cook until wilted.
- Whisk egg whites with salt and pepper, then pour over the vegetables.
- Cook until the omelette is set, then fold and serve.

BANANA AND PEANUT BUTTER SMOOTHIE

Time Required: 5 Minutes

Servings: 1

Ingredients:

- 1 banana
- 1 tablespoon peanut butter
- 1 cup almond milk
- Ice cubes

Instructions:

- Combine all ingredients in a blender.
- Blend until smooth.
- Pour into a glass and enjoy.

QUINOA BREAKFAST BOWL

Time Required: 20 Minutes

Servings: 1

Ingredients:

- 1/2 cup cooked quinoa
- 1/4 cup low-fat cottage cheese
- 1/4 cup diced apple
- 1 tablespoon honey
- Cinnamon to taste

Instructions:

- In a bowl, mix cooked quinoa with cottage cheese.
- Add diced apple and a sprinkle of cinnamon.
- Drizzle with honey before serving.

VEGGIE BREAKFAST WRAP

**Time Required:
15 Minutes**

____

Servings: 1

Ingredients:

- 1 whole-grain tortilla
- 1/4 cup bell peppers, diced
- 1/4 cup onions, diced
- 1/4 cup tomatoes, diced
- 1/4 cup spinach, chopped
- 2 egg whites
- Salt and pepper to taste

Instructions:

- Sauté bell peppers and onions in a non-stick pan until soft.
- Add tomatoes and spinach, cooking until spinach is wilted.
- Whisk egg whites with salt and pepper, then add to the pan.
- Cook until the eggs are set, then place the mixture on the tortilla.
- Roll up the tortilla and serve.

COTTAGE CHEESE AND PINEAPPLE BOWL

**Time Required:
5 Minutes**

____

Servings: 1

Ingredients:

- 1/2 cup low-fat cottage cheese
- 1/2 cup pineapple, diced
- 1 tablespoon sunflower seeds

Instructions:

- 1. In a bowl, combine cottage cheese and pineapple.
- Top with sunflower seeds before serving.

WHOLE-GRAIN PANCAKES WITH FRUIT

**Time Required:
20 Minutes**

____

Servings: 2

Ingredients:

- 1 cup whole-grain pancake mix
- 3/4 cup water
- 1/2 cup mixed fruit (sliced bananas, berries)
- Maple syrup (optional)

Instructions:

- Prepare the pancake batter according to package instructions using water.
- Cook pancakes on a non-stick pan until golden brown.
- Serve with mixed fruit and a drizzle of maple syrup if desired.

COTTAGE CHEESE AND PINEAPPLE BOWL

**Time Required:
10 Minutes**

____

Servings: 1

Ingredients:

- 1 slice whole-grain bread
- 1/2 cup low-sodium baked beans
- Fresh parsley for garnish

Instructions:

- Toast the bread to your liking.
- Warm the baked beans in a saucepan or microwave.
- Spoon the beans over the toast.
- Garnish with fresh parsley and serve.

LAUNCH RECIPES

GRILLED CHICKEN SALAD

**Time Required:
20 Minutes**

____

Servings: 2

Ingredients:

- 2 boneless, skinless chicken breasts
- 4 cups mixed greens
- 1 cup cherry tomatoes, halved
- 1/2 cucumber, sliced
- 1/4 red onion, thinly sliced
- 2 tablespoons balsamic vinaigrette

Instructions:

- Grill chicken breasts until fully cooked and let them rest.
- Slice chicken into strips.
- Toss mixed greens, tomatoes, cucumber, and onion in a large bowl.
- Top with chicken strips and drizzle with balsamic vinaigrette.

LENTIL SOUP

**Time Required:
45 Minutes**

____

Servings: 4

Ingredients:

- 1 cup lentils, rinsed
- 4 cups vegetable broth
- 1 carrot, diced
- 1 celery stalk, diced
- 1 onion, diced
- 2 garlic cloves, minced
- 1 teaspoon thyme
- Salt and pepper to taste

Instructions:

- In a pot, sauté onion, carrot, and celery until soft.
- Add garlic and cook for another minute.
- Pour in vegetable broth and lentils.
- Bring to a boil, then simmer until lentils are tender.
- Season with thyme, salt, and pepper.

TURKEY AND AVOCADO WRAP

**Time Required:
10 Minutes**

Servings: 1

Ingredients:

- 1 whole-grain tortilla
- 3 slices of turkey breast
- 1/2 ripe avocado, sliced
- 1/2 cup lettuce, shredded
- 1/4 cup tomato, diced
- Mustard to taste

Instructions:

- Lay the tortilla flat and spread mustard to taste.
- Layer turkey, avocado, lettuce, and tomato.
- Roll the tortilla tightly and cut in half.

QUINOA AND BLACK BEAN SALAD

**Time Required:
30 Minutes**

Servings: 2

Ingredients:

- 1 cup cooked quinoa
- 1 can black beans, drained and rinsed
- 1 red bell pepper, diced
- 1/4 cup fresh cilantro, chopped
- 2 tablespoons lime juice
- Salt and pepper to taste

Instructions:

- In a bowl, combine quinoa, black beans, and bell pepper.
- Add lime juice, cilantro, salt, and pepper.
- Toss to combine and serve chilled or at room temperature.

VEGGIE STIR-FRY WITH TOFU

**Time Required:
20 Minutes**

Servings: 2

Ingredients:

- 1 block firm tofu, drained and cubed
- 2 cups mixed vegetables (broccoli, bell peppers, carrots)
- 1 tablespoon soy sauce
- 1 teaspoon sesame oil
- 1 garlic clove, minced
- 1 teaspoon ginger, grated

Instructions:

- Heat sesame oil in a pan over medium heat.
- Add tofu and cook until golden brown.
- Add vegetables, garlic, and ginger, stir-frying until tender-crisp.
- Drizzle with soy sauce and serve.

MEDITERRANEAN CHICKPEA SALAD

**Time Required:
15 Minutes**

Servings: 2

Ingredients:

- 1 can chickpeas, drained and rinsed
- 1/2 cup cucumber, diced
- 1/2 cup tomatoes, diced
- 1/4 cup red onion, finely chopped
- 1/4 cup feta cheese, crumbled
- 2 tablespoons olive oil
- 1 tablespoon lemon juice
- Salt and pepper to taste

Instructions:

- In a bowl, combine chickpeas, cucumber, tomatoes, and onion.
- Add feta cheese, olive oil, lemon juice, salt, and pepper.
- Toss gently and serve.

BAKED SALMON WITH STEAMED VEGETABLES

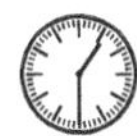

**Time Required:
30 Minutes**

Servings: 2

Ingredients:

- 2 salmon fillets
- 1 lemon, sliced
- 2 cups mixed vegetables (zucchini, green beans, carrots)
- Salt and pepper to taste

Instructions:

- Preheat oven to 375°F (190°C).
- Season salmon with salt and pepper, top with lemon slices.
- Bake for 20 minutes or until cooked through.
- Steam vegetables until tender.
- Serve salmon with steamed vegetables on the side.

CAPRESE SALAD WITH BALSAMIC GLAZE

**Time Required:
10 Minutes**

Servings: 2

Ingredients:

- 2 large tomatoes, sliced
- 1 ball fresh mozzarella cheese, sliced
- Fresh basil leaves
- Balsamic glaze
- Salt and pepper to taste

Instructions:

- Alternate layers of tomato and mozzarella slices on a plate.
- Tuck basil leaves between the layers.
- Drizzle with balsamic glaze.
- Season with salt and pepper.

SWEET POTATO AND BLACK BEAN BURRITO BOWL

Time Required: 40 Minutes

Servings: 2

Ingredients:

- 1 sweet potato, cubed
- 1 can black beans, drained and rinsed
- 1 cup brown rice, cooked
- 1/2 cup corn
- 1/4 cup salsa
- 1/4 cup low-fat Greek yogurt

Instructions:

- Roast sweet potato cubes at 400°F (200°C) for 25 minutes.
- In a bowl, layer brown rice, black beans, roasted sweet potato, and corn.
- Top with salsa and a dollop of Greek yogurt.

ZUCCHINI NOODLES WITH PESTO

Time Required: 15 Minutes

Servings: 2

Ingredients:

- 2 zucchinis, spiralized
- 1/4 cup pesto sauce
- Cherry tomatoes for garnish
- Parmesan cheese, grated (optional)

Instructions:

- Toss zucchini noodles with pesto sauce until well coated.
- Serve topped with cherry tomatoes and a sprinkle of Parmesan cheese if desired.

DINNER RECIPES

BAKED HERB-CRUSTED COD

**Time Required:
25 Minutes**

Servings: 2

Ingredients:

- 2 cod fillets
- 1/4 cup whole-wheat breadcrumbs
- 1 tablespoon fresh parsley, chopped
- 1 teaspoon olive oil
- 1 lemon, zest and juice
- Salt and pepper to taste

Instructions:

- Preheat oven to 400°F (200°C).
- Mix breadcrumbs, parsley, lemon zest, salt, and pepper.
- Brush cod with olive oil and lemon juice.
- Coat cod with breadcrumb mixture.
- Bake for 15-20 minutes or until flaky.

VEGETABLE STIR-FRY WITH BROWN RICE

**Time Required:
30 Minutes**

Servings: 2

Ingredients:

- 1 cup brown rice, cooked
- 2 cups mixed vegetables (broccoli, bell pepper, carrots)
- 1 tablespoon low-sodium soy sauce
- 1 teaspoon sesame oil
- 1 garlic clove, minced

Instructions:

- Heat sesame oil in a pan over medium heat.
- Add garlic and vegetables, stir-fry until tender.
- Add soy sauce and cooked rice, stir to combine.
- Serve hot.

GRILLED TURKEY BURGER

**Time Required:
20 Minutes**

____

Servings: 2

Ingredients:

- 1/2 pound ground turkey breast
- 1/4 cup onion, finely chopped
- 1 tablespoon Worcestershire sauce
- 2 whole-wheat burger buns
- Lettuce, tomato, and mustard for serving

Instructions:

- Combine turkey, onion, and Worcestershire sauce.
- Form into patties and grill until cooked through.
- Serve on buns with lettuce, tomato, and mustard.

LENTIL AND VEGETABLE STEW

**Time Required:
45 Minutes**

____

Servings: 4

Ingredients:

- 1 cup lentils
- 4 cups low-sodium vegetable broth
- 1 cup diced tomatoes
- 1 cup carrots, diced
- 1 cup celery, diced
- 1 onion, diced
- 2 garlic cloves, minced
- 1 teaspoon thyme

Instructions:

- In a pot, sauté onion, carrots, and celery.
- Add garlic, tomatoes, lentils, broth, and thyme.
- Simmer until lentils are tender.
- Serve warm.

ROASTED CHICKEN WITH VEGETABLES

Time Required: 1 hour

Servings: 4

Ingredients:

- 4 chicken breasts, skinless
- 2 cups mixed vegetables (zucchini, bell peppers, onions)
- 1 tablespoon olive oil
- 1 teaspoon rosemary
- Salt and pepper to taste

Instructions:

- 1. Preheat oven to 375°F (190°C).
- Season chicken with rosemary, salt, and pepper.
- Toss vegetables with olive oil and seasoning.
- Roast chicken and vegetables for 45 minutes.

SPAGHETTI SQUASH WITH MARINARA SAUCE

Time Required: 1 hour

Servings: 2

Ingredients:

- 1 spaghetti squash
- 1 cup marinara sauce
- 1/4 cup grated Parmesan cheese
- Fresh basil for garnish

Instructions:

- Cut squash in half, remove seeds, and bake face down at 400°F (200°C) for 40 minutes.
- Scrape squash strands into a bowl.
- Heat marinara sauce and pour over squash.
- Top with Parmesan and basil.

GRILLED VEGETABLE KABOBS

**Time Required:
30 minutes**

____

Servings: 2

Ingredients:

- 1 zucchini, cut into chunks
- 1 bell pepper, cut into chunks
- 1 red onion, cut into chunks
- 1 tablespoon olive oil
- 1 tablespoon balsamic vinegar
- Salt and pepper to taste

Instructions:

- Preheat grill to medium-high heat.
- Thread vegetables onto skewers.
- Brush with olive oil and balsamic vinegar.
- Grill until charred and tender.

CAULIFLOWER FRIED RICE

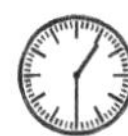

**Time Required:
20 minutes**

____

Servings: 2

Ingredients:

- 1 spaghetti squash
- 1 cup marinara sauce
- 1/4 cup grated Parmesan cheese
- Fresh basil for garnish

Instructions:

- Heat sesame oil in a pan.
- Add vegetables and cook until soft.
- Add cauliflower and soy sauce, cook for 5 minutes.
- Push mixture to the side, add eggs, and scramble.
- Mix everything together and serve.

CHICKPEA AND SPINACH CURRY

Time Required: 30 minutes

Servings: 4

Ingredients:

- 1 can chickpeas, drained and rinsed
- 4 cups spinach, washed
- 1 onion, diced
- 2 garlic cloves, minced
- 1 tablespoon curry powder
- 1 cup coconut milk
- Salt to taste

Instructions:

- Sauté onion and garlic until soft.
- Add curry powder and cook for 1 minute.
- Add chickpeas and coconut milk, simmer for 10 minutes.
- Stir in spinach until wilted.
- Season with salt and serve.

TURKEY MEATLOAF

Time Required: 1 hour 15 minutes

Servings: 2

Ingredients:

- 1 pound ground turkey breast
- 1/2 cup oats
- 1/4 cup onion, finely chopped
- 1 egg, beaten
- 1/2 cup tomato sauce
- 1 teaspoon Worcestershire sauce
- Salt and pepper to taste

Instructions:

- Preheat oven to 350°F (175°C).
- Mix all ingredients except tomato sauce.
- Form into a loaf and place in a baking dish.
- Top with tomato sauce.
- Bake for 1 hour or until cooked through.

SNACKS
RECIPES

CARROT AND HUMMUS DIP

Time Required: 5 minutes

Servings: 2

Ingredients:

- 1 cup baby carrots
- 1/2 cup hummus

Instructions:

- Serve baby carrots with a side of hummus for dipping.

GREEK YOGURT WITH HONEY AND ALMONDS

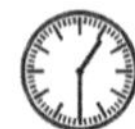

Time Required: 5 minutes

Servings: 1

Ingredients:

- 1 cup low-fat Greek yogurt
- 1 tablespoon honey
- 1 tablespoon almonds, slivered

Instructions:

- Top Greek yogurt with honey and slivered almonds.

APPLE SLICES WITH PEANUT BUTTER

**Time Required:
5 minutes**

—————————————

Servings: 1

Ingredients:

- 1 apple, cored and sliced
- 1 tablespoon natural peanut butter

Instructions:

- Spread peanut butter on apple slices.

RICE CAKES WITH AVOCADO

**Time Required:
5 minutes**

—————————————

Servings: 1

Ingredients:

- 2 rice cakes
- 1/2 avocado, mashed
- Salt and pepper to taste

Instructions:

- Spread mashed avocado on rice cakes.
- Season with salt and pepper.

CUCUMBER SANDWICHES

Time Required: 10 minutes

Servings: 2

Ingredients:

- 1 cucumber, sliced
- 1/4 cup low-fat cream cheese
- Fresh dill for garnish

Instructions:

- Spread cream cheese between two cucumber slices.
- Garnish with dill.

BAKED KALE CHIPS

Time Required: 20 minutes

Servings: 2

Ingredients:

- 1 bunch kale, torn into pieces
- 1 teaspoon olive oil
- Salt to taste

Instructions:

- Preheat oven to 300°F (150°C).
- Toss kale with olive oil and salt.
- Bake until crisp, about 15 minutes.

CHERRY TOMATOES WITH MOZZARELLA

**Time Required:
5 minutes**

———————————

Servings: 2

Ingredients:

- 1 cup cherry tomatoes, halved
- 1/2 cup mozzarella balls
- Balsamic glaze for drizzling

Instructions:

- Skewer tomato halves and mozzarella balls.
- Drizzle with balsamic glaze.

EDAMAME BEANS

**Time Required:
10 minutes**

———————————

Servings: 2

Ingredients:

- 1 cup edamame beans, shelled
- Sea salt to taste

Instructions:

- Steam or boil edamame until tender.
- Sprinkle with sea salt.

BANANA AND OATMEAL COOKIES

Time Required: 25 minutes

Servings: 4

Ingredients:

- 2 ripe bananas, mashed
- 1 cup rolled oats
- 1/4 cup dark chocolate chips

Instructions:

- Preheat oven to 350°F (175°C).
- Mix bananas, oats, and chocolate chips.
- Drop spoonfuls onto a baking sheet.
- Bake for 15 minutes.

ROASTED CHICKPEAS

Time Required: 40 minutes

Servings: 2

Ingredients:

- 1 can chickpeas, drained and rinsed
- 1 teaspoon olive oil
- 1/2 teaspoon paprika
- Salt to taste

Instructions:

- Preheat oven to 400°F (200°C).
- Toss chickpeas with olive oil, paprika, and salt.
- Roast until crispy, about 30 minutes.

DESSERTS RECIPES

MIXED BERRY SALAD

**Time Required:
10 minutes**

____

Servings: 2

Ingredients:

- 1 cup strawberries, hulled and halved
- 1 cup blueberries
- 1 cup raspberries
- 1 tablespoon honey
- Fresh mint leaves for garnish

Instructions:

- Combine all berries in a bowl.
- Drizzle with honey and gently toss.
- Garnish with mint leaves before serving.

BAKED APPLES WITH CINNAMON

**Time Required:
40 minutes**

____

Servings: 2

Ingredients:

- 4 apples, cored
- 2 teaspoons cinnamon
- 4 teaspoons honey

Instructions:

- Preheat oven to 350°F (175°C).
- Place apples in a baking dish.
- Fill each apple center with cinnamon and honey.
- Bake for 30-35 minutes until tender.

MANGO SORBET

**Time Required:
2 hours 15
minutes**

Servings: 4

Ingredients:

- 2 ripe mangoes, peeled and cubed
- 2 tablespoons honey
- 1 tablespoon lime juice

Instructions:

- Puree mangoes, honey, and lime juice until smooth.
- Freeze in a shallow dish for 2 hours, stirring every 30 minutes.
- Serve once it reaches a sorbet consistency.

PINEAPPLE AND COTTAGE CHEESE

**Time Required:
5 minutes**

Servings: 1

Ingredients:

- 1/2 cup low-fat cottage cheese
- 1/2 cup pineapple chunks

Instructions:

- Serve cottage cheese topped with pineapple chunks.

BANANA PUDDING PARFAIT

**Time Required:
15 minutes**

____

Servings: 2

Ingredients:

- 2 bananas, sliced
- 1 cup low-fat vanilla yogurt
- 1/4 cup granola

Instructions:

- Layer banana slices and yogurt in glasses.
- Top with granola before serving.

PEACH AND RASPBERRY CRISP

**Time Required:
50 minutes**

____

Servings: 4

Ingredients:

- 2 peaches, sliced
- 1 cup raspberries
- 1/2 cup rolled oats
- 2 tablespoons almond flour
- 2 tablespoons honey
- 1 teaspoon cinnamon

Instructions:

- Preheat oven to 375°F (190°C).
- Mix peaches and raspberries with 1 tablespoon honey and place in a baking dish.
- Combine oats, almond flour, cinnamon, and remaining honey to make the topping.
- Sprinkle topping over fruit.
- Bake for 30 minutes until golden.

CHOCOLATE-DIPPED STRAWBERRIES

**Time Required:
15 minutes**

Servings: 2

Ingredients:

- 1 cup strawberries
- 1/4 cup dark chocolate chips, melted

Instructions:

- Dip strawberries into melted chocolate.
- Place on a parchment-lined tray.
- Chill in the refrigerator until set.

COCONUT RICE PUDDING

**Time Required:
40 minutes**

Servings: 4

Ingredients:

- 1/2 cup rice, rinsed
- 2 cups coconut milk
- 1/4 cup honey
- 1 teaspoon vanilla extract

Instructions:

- Combine rice, coconut milk, and honey in a pot.
- Bring to a boil, then simmer until rice is tender.
- Stir in vanilla extract and serve warm or chilled.

POACHED PEARS IN SPICED TEA

**Time Required:
30 minutes**

Servings: 4

Ingredients:

- 4 pears, peeled
- 2 cups brewed spiced tea
- 2 tablespoons honey

Instructions:

- Combine tea and honey in a pot and bring to a simmer.
- Add pears and poach until tender.
- Serve pears with a drizzle of the poaching liquid.

YOGURT AND FRUIT POPSICLES

**Time Required:
4 hours**

Servings: 6

Ingredients:

- 2 cups low-fat Greek yogurt
- 1 cup mixed berries, pureed
- 2 tablespoons honey

Instructions:

- Mix yogurt, berry puree, and honey.
- Pour into popsicle molds.
- Freeze until solid, about 4 hours.

CONCLUSION

Upon concluding "No Gallbladder Diet Cookbook for Beginners," we pause to consider the path we have taken together. This book was more than simply a recipe book; it was a ray of light and direction for people just starting out in life without a gallbladder. We have discussed the value of a balanced diet, the changes your body goes through after a cholecystectomy, and the satisfaction that comes from cooking and enjoying meals that are tasty and gentle on your digestive tract throughout each chapter.

The meals were thoughtfully created with consideration for the dietary requirements and ease of digestion of those who do not have a gallbladder. Every meal, from hearty breakfasts to filling lunches, cosy dinners, and tasty snacks and sweets, is meant to satisfy without making you feel uncomfortable.

Recall that losing your gallbladder is a condition you must learn to live with, not a permanent diet of bland food and misery. You can keep eating tasty, nutrient-dense meals if you have the correct information and a selection of appropriate recipes. Allow this book to be your culinary partner, an inspiration when you're feeling stuck, and a constant reminder that you can still enjoy eating and be healthy.

I hope the "No Gallbladder Diet Cookbook for Beginners" proves the adaptability of our bodies and the resiliency of the human spirit. I look forward to many more dinners that feed the soul as well as the body. Salutations!